TAKE CONTROL OF YOUR HEART HEALTH:

Strategies for Preventing and Reversing Heart Disease

Janet martins

Contents

DISCLAIMER:

All content is provided as general information only, and should not be taken as medical advice or professional guidance. Please consult with a qualified healthcare provider if you have any questions or concerns about your individual situation.

INTRODUCTION

Heart disease is the leading cause of death in the United States for both men and women. However, it doesn't have to be this way! You can do many things to take control of your heart health and prevent or reverse heart disease. This book will discuss some of the most important strategies for preventing and reversing heart disease.

The first step to taking control of your heart health is understanding the risk factors for developing heart disease. These include high blood pressure, smoking, diabetes, obesity, physical inactivity, and an unhealthy diet. You should maintain a healthy weight through regular physical activity and a balanced diet to reduce these risk factors. Eating plenty of fruits and vegetables can help lower your cholesterol levels and reduce your risk for heart disease. Also, quitting or avoiding secondhand smoke protects your heart health.

Regularly monitoring your blood pressure and cholesterol levels is another important step in preventing or reversing heart disease.

PART 1

WHAT IS HEART DISEASE?

DEFINITION OF HEART DISEASE

Heart disease is any disorder that affects the heart. A number of different conditions, such as high blood pressure, smoking, diabetes, and other genetic factors can cause it. Unfortunately, heart disease is common in men and women of all ages and ethnicities. Although there is no single cause of heart disease, certain lifestyle choices and medical conditions can increase the risk.

TYPES OF HEART DISEASES

There are many types of heart disease, and each one has its symptoms and treatment. For some, lifestyle changes and medicine can make a huge difference in improving your health. For others, you may need surgery to make your ticker work well again.

Find out about some common types of heart disease, how to prevent them, and how they're treated.

Coronary Artery Disease (CAD)

CAD is the most common heart problem. With CAD, you may get blockages in your coronary arteries, which supply blood to your heart. That can lead to a decrease in the flow of blood to your heart muscle, keeping it from getting the oxygen it needs. The disease usually starts due to atherosclerosis, a condition sometimes called the hardening of the arteries.

Coronary heart disease can give you pain in your chest, called angina, or lead to a heart attack.

Some things that may put you at a higher risk of coronary artery disease are:

- Age (For men, the risk of heart disease goes up after age 55; for women, the risk rises sharply after menopause.)
- Being inactive
- Having diabetes or metabolic syndrome
- Family history of coronary heart disease
- Genetics
- High blood pressure
- High levels of LDL "bad" cholesterol or low levels of HDL "good" cholesterol
- Obesity
- Smoking
- Stress

Heart Arrhythmias

When you have an arrhythmia, your heart has an irregular beating pattern. Serious arrhythmias often develop from other heart problems but may also happen on their own.

Heart Failure

Heart failure occurs when your heart is unable to pump enough blood to meet your body's needs. While coronary artery disease is a common cause, it can also be the result of conditions like thyroid disease, high blood pressure, and cardiomyopathy.

Heart Valve Disease

Your heart is composed of four chambers and four valves that regulate the flow of blood between them and the lungs and blood vessels. A valve might experience difficulty opening and closing properly, leading to blockages or blood leakage. This can result in an irregular opening and shutting of the valve.

The causes of heart valve problems include infections such as rheumatic fever, congenital heart disease, high blood pressure, coronary artery disease, or as a result of a heart attack.

Diseases of the heart valves include:

- **Endocarditis.** This infection is usually caused by bacteria, which may enter the blood and take root in your heart during illness, after surgery, or after intravenous drugs. It often happens if you already have valve problems. Antibiotics can usually cure it, but the disease is life-threatening without treatment.

- If your heart valves are seriously damaged as a result of endocarditis, you may need valve replacement surgery.

- **Rheumatic heart disease.** This condition develops when your heart muscle and valves are damaged by rheumatic fever, which is linked to strep throat and scarlet fever.

- Rheumatic heart disease was more common earlier in the 20th century. But doctors are now able to prevent it by using antibiotics to treat the diseases that lead to it. If you get it, the symptoms usually appear many years after the infection.

Pericardial Disease

A disease affecting the pericardium, the sac surrounding the heart, is known as pericardial disease. One of the common types of pericardial disease is pericarditis, which is caused by viral infections, inflammatory conditions like lupus or rheumatoid arthritis, or damage to the pericardium. Pericarditis sometimes occurs after open heart surgery.

Cardiomyopathy (Heart Muscle Disease)

Cardiomyopathy is a condition where your heart muscle, or myocardium, becomes stretched, thickened, or rigid. This can cause your heart to become too weak to function properly. The causes of the disease can include:

- Genetic heart conditions.
- Reactions to certain drugs or toxins (like alcohol).
- Infections from a virus.
- Even chemotherapy.

However, in many cases, doctors cannot determine the exact cause.

Congenital Heart Disease

Congenital heart disease is a condition that occurs during fetal development, where the heart forms incorrectly. This can result in immediate problems at birth or may not show any symptoms until adulthood.

One of the most frequently occurring congenital heart problems is septal abnormalities, which are holes in the wall between the left and right sides of the heart. You can undergo a procedure to repair the hole.

Pulmonary stenosis is a type of abnormality that occurs when a narrow valve reduces blood flow to the lungs. It can be treated by either opening or replacing the valve through a medical procedure or surgery. In certain cases, babies may have an open ductus arteriosus after birth, causing blood to leak back into the pulmonary artery and put a strain on the heart. This can be treated through medication or surgery.

CAUSES AND RISK FACTORS FOR HEART DISEASE

Heart disease symptoms depend on the type of heart disease.

Symptoms of heart disease in the blood vessels

Coronary artery disease is a common heart condition that affects the major blood vessels that supply the heart muscle. Cholesterol deposits (plaques) in the heart arteries usually cause coronary artery disease. The buildup of these plaques is called atherosclerosis (ath-ur-o-skluh-ROE-sis). Atherosclerosis reduces blood flow to the heart and other parts of the body. It can lead to a heart attack, chest pain (angina), or stroke.

The symptoms of coronary artery disease may vary in men and women. For example, men often experience chest pain, while women may have additional symptoms like shortness of breath, nausea, extreme fatigue, and chest discomfort.

Symptoms of coronary artery disease can include:

- Chest pain, chest tightness, chest pressure, and chest discomfort (angina)
- Shortness of breath
- Pain in the neck, jaw, throat, upper belly area, or back
- Pain, numbness, weakness, or coldness in the legs or arms if the blood vessels in those body areas are narrowed

It's possible to have coronary artery disease without being diagnosed until after experiencing a heart attack, stroke, angina, or heart failure. To detect heart problems early, monitoring for heart symptoms and discussing any concerns with your healthcare provider is important. Regular health checkups can also help identify cardiovascular disease in its early stages.

Heart disease symptoms caused by irregular heartbeats (heart arrhythmias)

The heart may beat too quickly, too slowly, or irregularly. Heart arrhythmia symptoms can include:

- Chest pain or discomfort
- Dizziness
- Fainting (syncope) or near fainting
- Fluttering in the chest
- Lightheadedness
- Racing heartbeat (tachycardia)
- Shortness of breath

- Slow heartbeat (bradycardia)

Heart disease symptoms caused by congenital heart defects

Serious congenital heart defects usually are noticed soon after birth. Congenital heart defect symptoms in children could include:

- Pale gray or blue skin or lips (cyanosis)
- Swelling in the legs, belly area, or areas around the eyes
- In an infant, shortness of breath during feedings leads to poor weight gain

Less serious congenital heart defects are often not diagnosed until later in childhood or adulthood.

Symptoms of congenital heart defects that usually aren't immediately life-threatening include:

- Easily getting short of breath during exercise or activity
- Easily tiring during exercise or activity
- Swelling of the hands, ankles, or feet

Heart disease symptoms caused by diseased heart muscle (cardiomyopathy)

Early stages of cardiomyopathy may not cause noticeable symptoms. As the condition worsens, symptoms may include:

- Dizziness, lightheadedness, and fainting
- Fatigue
- Feeling short of breath during activity or at rest
- Feeling short of breath at night when trying to sleep or waking up short of breath
- Irregular heartbeats that feel rapid pounding or fluttering
- Swollen legs, ankles, or feet

Heart disease symptoms caused by heart valve problems (valvular heart disease)

The heart has four valves aortic, mitral, pulmonary, and tricuspid. They open and close to move blood through the heart. Many things can damage the heart valves. A heart valve may become narrowed (stenosis), leaky (regurgitation or insufficiency), or close improperly (prolapse).

Valvular heart disease is also called heart valve disease. Depending on which valve isn't **working properly, heart valve disease symptoms generally include the following:**

- Chest pain
- Fainting (syncope)
- Fatigue
- Irregular heartbeat
- Shortness of breath
- Swollen feet or ankles

Endocarditis is an infection that affects the heart valves and inner lining of the heart chambers and heart valves (endocardium).

Endocarditis symptoms can include:

- Dry or persistent cough
- Fever

- Heartbeat changes
- Shortness of breath
- Skin rashes or unusual spots
- Swelling of the legs or belly area
- Weakness or fatigue

Causes

Heart disease causes depend on the specific type of heart disease. There are many different types of heart disease.

Understanding the causes of heart disease may help to understand how the heart works.

- The heart is divided into two upper chambers (atria) and two lower chambers (ventricles).
- The right side of the heart moves blood to the lungs through blood vessels (pulmonary arteries).

- The blood picks up oxygen in the lungs and then returns to the left side of the heart through the pulmonary veins.

- The left side of the heart pumps the blood through the aorta and out to the rest of the body.

Heart valves

Four heart valves are in charge of directing blood flow: the aortic, mitral, pulmonary, and tricuspid valves. These valves have a one-way opening mechanism and open only when necessary. To ensure no leakage, the valves must fully open and tightly close.

Heartbeats

A beating heart squeezes (contracts) and relaxes in a continuous cycle.

- During contraction (systole), the lower heart chambers (ventricles) squeeze tight.

This action forces blood to the lungs and the rest of the body.

- During relaxation (diastole), the ventricles fill with blood from the upper heart chambers (atria).

Electrical system

The heart's electrical system keeps it beating. The heartbeat controls the continuous exchange of oxygen-rich blood with oxygen-poor blood. This exchange keeps you alive.

- Electrical signals start in the upper right chamber (right atrium).
- The signals travel through specialized pathways to the lower heart chambers (ventricles). This tells the heart to pump.

CAUSES OF CORONARY ARTERY DISEASE

Coronary artery disease is commonly caused by atherosclerosis, the accumulation of fatty plaques in the arteries. Risk factors such as poor diet, lack of exercise, obesity, and smoking can increase the likelihood of developing this condition. Therefore, making healthy lifestyle choices can be beneficial in reducing the risk of atherosclerosis.

Causes of irregular heartbeats (arrhythmias)

Common causes of arrhythmias or conditions that can lead to them include:

- Cardiomyopathy
- Coronary artery disease
- Diabetes
- Drug misuse
- Emotional stress
- Excessive use of alcohol or caffeine
- Heart problem present at birth (congenital heart defects)
- High blood pressure
- Smoking

- Heart valve disease

- Use of certain medications, including those bought without a prescription, and herbs and supplements

Causes of congenital heart defects

A congenital heart defect is a condition that affects the baby's heart development in the womb, occurring about a month after conception. It alters the normal flow of blood in the heart. Certain medical factors, genes, and medication can increase the likelihood of such defects.

Causes of a thickened or enlarged heart muscle (cardiomyopathy)

The cause of cardiomyopathy depends on the type:

- **Dilated cardiomyopathy.** The cause of this most common type of cardiomyopathy often is unknown. It may be passed down through families (inherited). Dilated cardiomyopathy typically starts in the heart's main pumping chamber (left ventricle). Many things can cause damage to the left ventricle, including heart attacks, infections, toxins, and some drugs, including cancer medicines.

- **Hypertrophic cardiomyopathy.** This type is usually passed down through families (inherited).

- **Restrictive cardiomyopathy.** This is the least common type of cardiomyopathy. It can occur for no known reason. Sometimes it's caused by a buildup of protein called amyloid in the heart (cardiac amyloidosis) or connective tissue disorders.

Causes of heart infection

A heart infection, such as endocarditis, occurs when germs reach the heart or valves. The most common causes of heart infections are:

- Bacteria
- Viruses
- Parasites

Causes of heart valve disease

Many things can cause diseases of the heart valve. For example, some people are born with heart valve disease (congenital heart valve disease). In addition, heart valve disease may also be caused by conditions such as:

- Rheumatic fever
- Infections (infectious endocarditis)
- Connective tissue disorders

*****

RISK FACTORS

Risk factors for heart disease include:

- **Age.** Growing older increases the risk of damaged and narrowed arteries and weakened or thickened heart muscle.

- **Sex.** Men are generally at greater risk of heart disease. The risk for women increases after menopause.

- **Family history.** A family history of heart disease increases the risk of coronary artery disease, especially if a parent developed it early (before age 55 for a male relative, such as your brother or father, and 65 for a female relative, such as your mother or sister).

- **Smoking.** If you smoke, quit. Substances in tobacco smoke damage the arteries. Heart attacks are more common in smokers than in nonsmokers. If you need help quitting, talk to your healthcare provider about strategies that can help.

- **Unhealthy diet.** Diets high in fat, salt, sugar, and cholesterol have been linked to heart disease.

- **High blood pressure.** Uncontrolled high blood pressure can cause the arteries to become hard and thick. These changes interrupt blood flow to the heart and body.

- **High cholesterol.** Having high cholesterol increases the risk of atherosclerosis. Atherosclerosis has been linked to heart attacks and strokes.

- **Diabetes.** Diabetes increases the risk of heart disease. Obesity and high blood pressure increase the risk of diabetes and heart disease.

- **Obesity.** Excess weight typically worsens other heart disease risk factors.

- **Lack of exercise.** Being inactive (a sedentary lifestyle) is associated with many forms of heart disease and some of its risk factors.

- **Stress.** Unrelieved stress may damage the arteries and worsen other risk factors for heart disease.

- **Poor dental health.** It's important to brush and floss your teeth and gums often. Also, get regular dental checkups. Unhealthy teeth and gums make it easier for germs to enter the bloodstream and travel to the heart. This can cause endocarditis.

COMPLICATIONS

Complications of heart disease include:

- **Heart failure.** This is one of the most common complications of heart disease.

Heart failure occurs when the heart can't pump enough blood to meet the body's needs.

- **Heart attack.** A heart attack may occur if a blood clot is stuck in a blood vessel that goes to the heart.

- **Stroke.** The risk factors that lead to heart disease can also lead to an ischemic stroke. This type of stroke happens when the arteries to the brain are narrowed or blocked. Too little blood reaches the brain. A stroke is a medical emergency — brain tissue begins to die within just a few minutes of a stroke.

- **Aneurysm.** An aneurysm is a bulge in the wall of an artery. If an aneurysm bursts, you may have life-threatening internal bleeding.

- **Peripheral artery disease.** In this condition, the arms or legs — usually the legs — don't get enough blood. This causes symptoms, most notably leg pain when walking (claudication). Atherosclerosis can lead to peripheral artery disease.

- **Sudden cardiac arrest.** Sudden cardiac arrest is the sudden loss of heart function, breathing, and consciousness. It's usually due to a problem with the heart's electrical system. Sudden cardiac arrest is a medical emergency. If not treated immediately, it results in sudden cardiac death.

PART 2

HOW TO PREVENT AND TREAT HEART DISEASE

Treatment for heart disease varies by condition and severity. For example, coronary artery disease can be treated with lifestyle changes or medication, while a serious heart rhythm problem may need an implantable device, like a pacemaker.

Your doctor will devise a treatment plan that is best for your needs. Make sure to follow directions carefully and fully.

Generally, heart disease treatment can include:

Lifestyle Modifications These are often the first steps to managing heart disease. Lifestyle changes include eating a heart-healthy diet low in sodium and fat, exercising regularly, quitting smoking, and limiting alcohol use.

Medication When lifestyle changes are not enough, your doctor may prescribe medication to treat heart disease. The type of drug prescribed will depend on the condition and severity.

Medications commonly used in the treatment of heart disease can include:

- Anticoagulants, or blood thinners, that decrease the blood clotting ability are used to treat certain blood vessels, heart, and heart rhythm conditions. These drugs help prevent harmful blood clots from forming in the blood vessels or heart and may prevent clots from becoming larger and causing more serious problems. Angiotensin-converting enzyme (ACE) inhibitors expand blood vessels and decrease resistance by lowering levels of hormones that regulate blood pressure, allowing blood to flow through the body more easily. Beta-blockers work by slowing the heart rate and decreasing the effects of adrenaline on the heart. This helps lower blood pressure, so the heart has to do less work. Calcium channel blockers interrupt the movement of calcium into the blood vessels and heart cells. This medication can relax the blood vessels and lower the heart rate. Digitalis can help the heart contract harder when its pumping function has been weakened.

Diuretics, also known as water pills, rid the body of excess fluids and sodium through urination, helping to relieve the heart's workload. These pills also decrease the backup of fluid in the lungs and other parts of the body, like ankles and legs. Cholesterol-lowering medicines, like statins, decrease LDL (the "bad") cholesterol levels in the blood.

Surgery If lifestyle changes and medication are not enough, surgery may be needed. The type of heart disease you have and how much damage has been done to your heart will determine which procedure your doctor recommends.

Medical procedures to treat heart disease can include:

- Angioplasty is a procedure that involves special tubing with an attached deflated balloon that is threaded up to the coronary artery. The balloon is inflated to widen the blocked areas where blood flow to the heart has been slowed or cut off. Stent placement involves a wire mesh tube, called a stent, that prop opens an artery during angioplasty and stays in the artery permanently. Bypass surgery treats blocked arteries by removing arteries or veins from other parts of the body and using them to reroute blood around arteries that are clogged to improve blood flow to the heart. Radiofrequency ablation is used to treat various heart rhythm problems when drugs are ineffective. It involves a catheter with an electrode at its tip guided through the veins to the heart muscle. The catheter is placed at the exact site in the heart where electrical signals stimulate the abnormal heart rhythm, and mild radiofrequency energy is transmitted to the pathway, destroying selected cells in a very small area. A heart transplant is performed in very serious circumstances when a heart is irreversibly damaged. The procedure involves removing a diseased heart and replacing it with a healthy one from an organ donor.

TIPS FOR PREVENTING HEART DISEASE

Eat a healthy diet.

Maintaining a heart-healthy diet is key to preventing heart disease. The American Heart Association (AHA) recommends the Dietary Approaches to Stop Hypertension (DASH) eating plan for optimal heart health. The DASH diet focuses on heart-healthy foods that are low in fat, cholesterol, and sodium and rich in nutrients, protein, and fiber. Foods to focus on include fruits and vegetables, whole grains, fat-free or low-fat dairy products, fish, poultry, and nuts. In addition, the DASH eating plan limits red meats, sweets, added sugars, and sugar-sweetened beverages.

Exercise regularly.

Physical activity has numerous benefits, including strengthening your heart and improving circulation. For optimal heart health, the AHA recommends at least 30 minutes of moderate-intensity aerobic activity five days a week or at least 25 minutes of vigorous aerobic activity three days a week in addition to moderate- to high-intensity muscle-strengthening activity two days a week.

Control your blood pressure.

High blood pressure is one of the biggest risk factors for heart disease. Be sure to get tested regularly for high blood pressure. That means once a year for most adults and more often as directed if your blood pressure is high. According to the AHA, a normal blood pressure reading is 120/80 millimeters of mercury (mmHg). Once you get above this range, your risk of cardiovascular disease increases. Lifestyle changes and medication can help lower blood pressure.

Keep cholesterol under control.

High cholesterol can clog your arteries and raise your risk of coronary artery disease and heart attack. So again, your doctor will prescribe lifestyle changes and medication, if needed, to lower your cholesterol.

Maintain a healthy weight.

Being overweight or obese significantly increases the risk of heart disease since it raises the risk of other heart disease risk factors, including high blood pressure, high cholesterol, and diabetes. Controlling weight through a healthy diet and exercise will help prevent these conditions and lower your risk of heart disease.

Limit alcohol intake.

Too much alcohol can raise your blood pressure and add extra calories to your diet, which can lead to weight gain, both of which increase the risk of heart disease. Healthy women of all ages and men older than 65 should stick to drinking up to one drink a day, while men 65 and younger should limit their alcohol intake to two drinks a day. One drink equals 12 ounces of beer, 5 ounces of wine, or 1 ½ ounces of liquor.

Don't smoke.

If you use tobacco, it is important to quit. If you don't smoke, it is important not to start. Smoking cigarettes raises your blood pressure and increases your heart attack and stroke risk. Talk to your doctor about methods to quit that will work best for you.

Manage stress.

Stress can affect the heart in all sorts of ways, including raising blood pressure and, in extreme cases, even triggering a heart attack. Additionally, some people cope with stress in unhealthy ways, such as overeating or turning to alcohol or tobacco, which increases the risk of heart disease. Healthy stress management methods include exercise, meditation, and cognitive behavioral therapy.

Manage diabetes.

Having diabetes significantly increases your risk for heart disease because, over time, high blood sugar can damage your blood vessels. So get screened for diabetes regularly, and if you have the condition, follow your doctor's guidance to keep it under control.

CONCLUSION

Heart disease is a major health concern, but it doesn't have to be. Taking small steps today can go a long way in preventing heart problems in the future. Eating a healthy diet, exercising regularly, and avoiding smoking and excessive alcohol consumption are all important strategies for maintaining good cardiovascular health. Additionally, seeing your healthcare provider regularly for check-ups and taking any prescribed medications can help keep your heart healthy. Dedication and effort can reduce your risk of developing heart disease and help you stay healthy!

Take charge of your well-being today - start making small changes that will lead to big rewards in the future! It may take some time to adjust to healthier habits, but with perseverance and commitment, you'll be on your way to a healthier and happier life. So start today and make sure that your heart is strong for many years to come!